CLASS

DRUGS

**INCLUDING DOSAGES
(PHARMACOLOGY)**

SIXTH EDITION

Narinder Dev

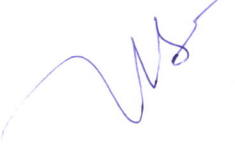

JAYPEE BROTHERS
MEDICAL PUBLISHERS (P) LTD
New Delhi

Published by

Jitendar P Vij

Jaypee Brothers Medical Publishers (P) Ltd

B-3 EMCA House, 23/23B Ansari Road, Daryaganj, **New Delhi** 110 002, India
Phones: +91-11-23272143, +91-11-23272703, +91-11-23282021, +91-11-23245672,
Rel: 32558559, Fax: +91-11-23276490, +91-11-23245683
e-mail: jaypee@jaypeebrothers.com, Visit our website: www.jaypeebrothers.com

Classification of Drugs

© 2007, Narinder Dev

All rights reserved. No part of this publication should be reproduced, stored in a retrieval system, or transmitted in any form or by any means: electronic, mechanical, photocopying, recording, or otherwise, without the prior written permission of the author and the publisher.

> This book has been published in good faith that the material provided by author is original. Every effort is made to ensure accuracy of material, but the publisher, printer and author will not be held responsible for any inadvertent error(s). In case of any dispute, all legal matters are to be settled under Delhi jurisdiction only.

Sixth Edition : 2007
Reprint : **2008**
ISBN 81-8448-106-3

Typeset at JPBMP typesetting unit
Printed at Rajkamal Electric Press, G.T.Karnal Road, Industrial Area, Delhi-33

PREFACE TO THE SIXTH EDITION

As a periodic affair, the book has been reviewed to remove errors whatsoever present. A few more chapters have also been added. Every possible effort has been made to provide correct dosages of all the medicines in clinical practice but in case of doubt, please consult the textbook.

I hope students will appreciate this comprehensive presentation of the subject.

Narinder Dev

PREFACE TO THE FIRST EDITION

It gives me pleasure in presenting this small booklet for medical students. This book has been formulated in a way to give precisely the various drugs and their dosages. The peculiar small size has been made to make the book handy for quick revision by students. I am thankful to various authors of standard books from whose publications help has been taken for compiling this book.

I hope students will find it useful.

1st September, 1978 **Narinder Dev**

Contents

Chapter I : Autonomic Nervous System ... 1–19
1. Parasympathomimetic ... 1
2. Sympathomimetic Drugs ... 3
3. Sympathetic (Adrenergic) Blocking Agents ... 12
4. Parasympatholytic Drugs ... 15
5. Ganglion Blocking Agents ... 17

Chapter II : Cardiovascular System ... 20–37
1. Drugs Influencing the Cardiac Rate ... 20
2. Anti-arrhythmic Drugs ... 22
3. Vasoconstrictors ... 26
4. Vasodilators ... 28
5. Hypotensive ... 31
6. Coronary Dilators ... 34

vi | *Classification of Drugs*

7. Drugs used in Peripheral Vascular Diseases	...	36
8. Drugs used in Atherosclerosis	...	36
Chapter III : Respiratory System	...	**38-46**
1. Bronchodilators	...	38
2. Respiratory Stimulants	...	39
3. Respiratory Depressants	...	41
4. Antitussive	...	42
5. Expectorants	...	44
Chapter IV: Drugs Acting on Gastrointestinal Tract	...	**47-60**
1. Bitters	...	47
2. Carminatives	...	48
3. Gastric Antacids	...	48
4. Digestants	...	49
5. Emetics	...	50
6. Antiemetics	...	51
7. Intestinal Spasmodics	...	54
8. Intestinal Antispasmodics	...	55
9. Purgatives	...	56
10. Intestinal Astringents	...	59

Contents | vii

Chapter V: Central Nervous System ... **61–83**
   1. Hypnotics ... 61
   2. Analgesics ... 65
   3. General Anaesthetics ... 69
   4. Anti-epileptic Drugs ... 71
   5. Pyretics ... 76
   6. Anti-pyretics ... 77
   7. CNS Stimulants ... 78
   8. Tranquilizers ... 80
   9. Anti-depressants ... 82
  10. Psychotogenic Drugs ... 83

Chapter VI: Drugs Acting on Urinary System ... **84–91**
   1. Diuretics ... 84
   2. Urinary Antiseptics ... 87
   3. Anti-diuretics ... 90

Chapter VII: Anti-histaminics ... **92–93**

Chapter VIII: Drugs Acting on Uterus ... **94–95**

Chapter IX: Drugs Acting on Eye ... **96–98**

Chapter X: Haemopoietic System ... **99–103**

viii | *Classification of Drugs*

Chapter XI: Drugs Used in Gout	...	**104–111**
Chapter XII: Endocrinology	...	**112–122**
Chapter XIII: Chemotherapy	...	**123–141**
1. Sulfonamides	...	123
2. Antibiotics	...	124
3. Antitubercular Drugs	...	129
4. Anti-leprosy Drugs	...	131
5. Drugs used for Syphilis	...	132
6. Anti-viral Drugs	...	133
7. Anti-neoplastic Drugs	...	134
8. Chemotherapy of Helminthic Infections	...	135

CHAPTER I
AUTONOMIC NERVOUS SYSTEM

1. Parasympathomimetic
Or
Cholinergic Drugs

1. *Choline esters*

   Act at all sites like acetylcholine
   - (i) Acetylcholine
   - (ii) Methacholine - 10 to 30 mg s/c
   - (iii) Carbachol – 0.2 to 0.5 mg s/c or 1 to 4 mg orally
   - (iv) Bethanechol – 2.5 mg s/c or 5 to 30 mg orally

2. *Naturally occuring alkaloids*

   Act selectively on end organs affected by acetylcholine
   - (i) Pilocarpine – 5-10 mg orally or parenterally. In ophthalmology 0.5-4% solution
   - (ii) Muscarine
   - (iii) Arecoline.

2 | Classification of Drugs

3. **A. Cholinesterase inhibitors (Reversible)**

   Inactivate the enzyme which destroys acetylcholine
   - (i) Physostigmine (Eserine) – 0.15 to 1% locally or 2 mg s/c
   - (ii) Neostigmine (Prostigmine) – 15 to 30 mg q.i.d. orally or 0.25 to 1.00 mg s/c
   - (iii) Pyridostigmine 1.5 mg s/c or 60-240 mg orally/day
   - (iv) Benzpyrinium
   - (v) Ambenonium (Mytelase) – 10 mg orally
   - (vi) Edrophonium – 3 mg/IV
   - (vii) Demecarium

   B. Cholinesterase inhibitors (Irreversible) or Organophosphorus compounds
   - (i) DFP (Di-isopropyl fluorophosphate) – 0.1% arachis oil for use in eye
   - (ii) HETP (Hexa ethyl tetra phosphate)
   - (iii) TEPP (Tetra ethyl pyrophosphate)
   - (iv) OMPA (Octa methyl pyrophosphoramide)

2. Sympathomimetic Drugs
Or
Adrenergic Drugs

A. Classification as per their chemical structure

1. *Catechol derivatives*
   — Adrenaline (1 : 1000) 0.2-0.5 ml s/c
   — Nor-drin (Nor-adrenaline) 4 µg/mt (I/V infusion)
   — Isopropyl nor-drin (Isoprenaline) 10 mg s/l for bronchial asthma. 5 µg/ml I/V for heart-block
   — Ethyl nor-drin
   — Dopamine 2.5 µg/kg/mt

2. *Phenol derivatives*
   — Phenylephrine — As mydriatic 1-2%,
        As nasal decongestant 0.25%
   — Metarminol
        Vaso pressor – 2.10 mg I/M or I/V
        Nasal decongestant – 0.25 – 0.5%

- Tyramine
- Hydroxyamphetamine
  - Nasal decongestant 1%
  - Stock Adams syndrome → 20-60 mg thrice a day orally
- Isoxsuprine
- Nylidrine

3. *Methoxybenzene derivatives*
   - Methoxamine
     - Vaso pressor – 5-30 mg I/M or I/V
     - Nasal decongestant – 0.5% solution
   - Methoxyphenamine.

4. *Benzene derivatives*
   - Ephedrine tablets – 15-60 mg
     Inj – 25-50 mg/ml
     Sol – 0.5 – 3.0%

Dosage:—
Bronchial asthma – 25-50 mg t.d.s. orally
Nasal decongestant 0.5-3.0%
To prevent hypotension during spinal anaesthesia 50 mg I/M or I/V

— Amphetamine → for narcolepsy 20-60 mg
(Dextroamphetamine)
— Methamphetamine
— Mephenteramine
  - Vaso pressor – 10-30 mg I/M or I/V
  - Nasal decongestant –0.5%
— Benzphetamine
— Phentermine.

5. *3, 5 Dihydrobenzene derivatives*
   — Orciprenaline
   — Terbutaline
   — Fenoterol.

6 | *Classification of Drugs*

6. ***Imidazoline derivatives***
   — Nephazoline
   — Tetrahydrozoline
   — Xylometazoline
   — Oxymetazoline

7. ***Alicyclic derivatives***

   — Cyclopentamine
   - Vaso pressor 25 mg I/M
   - Nasal decongestant – 0.5%

   — Propylhexedrine

B. **Classification as per their site and mode of action**

   1. ***Drugs acting directly on Adrenergic receptors***
      (a) *Alpha receptors*
      — Noradrenaline
      — Mephentermine
      — Metarminol

- Methoxamine
- Phenylephrine

(b) *Beta receptors*
- Isoprenaline
- Isoxsuprine
- Nylidrine

(c) *Acting both on α and β receptors*
- Adrenaline
- Ephedrine
- Amphetamine
- Paredrine.

2. ***Drugs acting indirectly by release of catecholamines at adrenergic nerve endings***
   - Amphetamine
   - Methamphetamine (Methadrin)
   - Mephentermine
   - Ephedrine

8 | Classification of Drugs

3. **Drugs acting by inhibiting Monoamine oxidase** (MAO)
   — Ephedrine
   — Amphetamine
4. **Drugs acting by inhibiting catechol – O-methyl transferase**
   — Pyragallol
   — Catechol.

Therapeutic classification or classification as per clinics use—

1. *Vasoconstrictor or Pressor agents*
   — Noradrenaline (Nor-epinephrine) 4 mg/litre I.V. fluid transfused at the rate of 4 µg/mt or 15-40 drops/mt
   — Phenylephrine – 0.5 mg I/V slowly or 5 mg s/c or I/M
   — Mephentermine (Wyamine) – 10-20 mg orally b.d. or t.d.s.

   Or

   15-30 mg I/M or I/V in transfusion fluid
   — Methoxamine (vasoxyl) – 5-20 mg I/M or 5-10 mg I/V

- Cyclopentamine (Clopane) – 10-25 mg I/V or I/M and 0.5-1% locally as nasal decongestant.
- Methamphetamine – 2.5-10.0 mg orally
- Metarminol (Aramine) 2-10 mg I/M or I/V 0.25-0.5% as nasal decongestant locally
- Hydroxyamphetamine – 1% as nasal decongestant, 20-60 mg t.d.s. or q.i.d. orally.

2. *Anti histaminics*
   - Adrenaline – 0.25-0.5 ml (1:1000 aquous sol.) s/c and 1:1000 or 1:10,000 solution locally for eye and E.N.T. problems
   - Orciprenaline – 20-60 mg/day.

3. *Nasal Decongestants*
   - Naphazoline – 0.05-0.1% Aquous isotonic solution
   - Phenylpropanolamine
   - Methoxamine (Vasoxyl) 0.5% sol.
   - Tuamine – 1% locally.

- Xylometazoline
- Phenylephrine 0.25%
- Clopane – 0.5-1% locally
- Propylhexedrine
- Hydroxyamphetamine – 1% locally
- Tetrahydrozoline – 1% solution locally
- Ephedrine – 0.5-2.0% locally.

4. *Bronchodilators*
   - Isoprenaline – 5.20 mg sublingually
   - Ephedrine – 25-50 mg t.d.s. or q.i.d. orally
   - Methoxyphenamine – 50-100 mg orally
   - Adrenaline 0.2-5.0 ml (1:1000 aquous sol) s/c Intracardiac in cases of cardiac arrest
   - Orciprenaline (Alupent) – 20-80 mg/day orally, 0.5-1.0 mg s/c or i/m
   - Salbutamol – 100 mcg. inhalation, 2-4 mg orally.

5. **Vasodilators or drugs used in Peripheral vascular disease:**
   - Isoxsuprine (Duvadilan) 10-40 mg/day orally

— Nylidrine (Arlidine) – 6-24 mg/day orally
Or
2.5-5 mg s/c or i/m.

6. *Corticomedullary stimulants*
   — Amphetamine (Benzedrene) – 5-10 mg orally/day
   — Dexamphetamine (Dexedrene for narcolepsy) 20-60 mg
   — Methamphetamine (Methedrene) – 2.5-5.0 mg orally t.d.s. as C.N.S. stimulant
   — Ephedrine – 15-60 mg orally per day.

7. *Anorexigenics*
   — Dexamphetamine
   — Methyl amphetamine
   — Amphetamine
   — Phenmetrazine.

8. *Cardiac stimulants*
   — Ephedrine
   — Isoprenaline
   — Hydroxyamphetamine.

12 | *Classification of Drugs*

9. ***Drugs used in Heart block***
   — Adrenaline
   — Isoprenaline – 5 µg/mt I/V infusion.
10. ***Drugs used in Paroxysmal atrial tachycardia***
    — Phenylephrine
    — Methoxamine.
11. ***Mydriatics***
    — Phenylephrine – 1-2% solution.

3. Sympathetic (Adrenergic) Blocking Agents

1. *Alpha adrenergic blocking agents*
   (a) *Natural alkaloids*

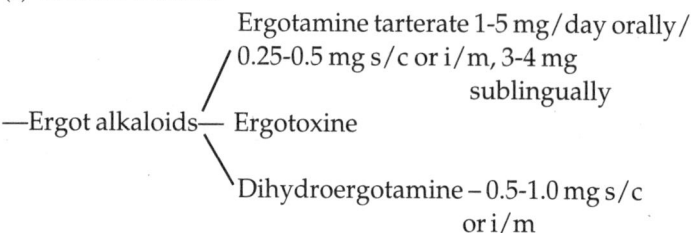

   —Ergot alkaloids
   - Ergotamine tarterate 1-5 mg/day orally / 0.25-0.5 mg s/c or i/m, 3-4 mg sublingually
   - Ergotoxine
   - Dihydroergotamine – 0.5-1.0 mg s/c or i/m

(b) *Imidazoline derivatives*
 — Tolazoline (Priscol) – 25 mg t.d.s.
 — Phentolamine (Regitine) – 5-30 mg i/m or i/v
(c) β *Haloalkyl amines*
 — Phenoxybenzamine (Dibenzyline) – 10-240 mg/day orally or 1 mg/kg/I/V infusion in 20 minutes
 — Dibenamine – 4-6 mg/kg body wt. not exceeding 100 mg single total dose
(d) *Benzodioxane derivatives*
 — Piperoxan – 15-20 mg I/V
 — Dibozane
(e) *Dibazapine derivatives*
 — Azapetine – 25-75 mg orally t.d.s.
       or 5-10 mg/kg i/v

(f) Miscellaneous — Yohimbine
                 — Chlorpromazine
                 — Phthalazines

2. **β–*adrenergic blocking agents***
 — Propranolol (Inderal) – 10-40 mg orally 6-8 hourly
 or 1-10 mg I/V slowly
 — Pronethalol
 — Dichlorisoprenaline
 — Dichloronoradrenaline
 — Dichloroadrenaline.
3. *Post ganglionic sympathetic nerve blocking agents (Adrenergic nerve blocking agents)*
 — Guanithidine (Ismelin) – 10-200 mg/day orally
 — Bethanidine (Esbatal) – 20-650 mg/day
  Guanoclor (Vatensol)
 — Methyl dopa – 0.5-2.5 gm/day orally
 — Reserpine (Serpasil) – 0.3-0.5 mg/day
 — M. A. O. inhibitors

4. Parasympatholytic Drugs
Or
Parasympathetic Blocking Agents
Or
Antimuscarinic Drugs
Or
Anticholinergic Drugs

The drugs which block the postganglionic parasympathetic nerves and thereby block the muscarinic action of acetylcholine other cholinomimetic drugs are known as parasympatholytic drugs.

Classification

A. *Natural alkaloids*

Belladona alkaloids (From Atropa Belladona, Dhatura, Stramonium and Hyoscyamin niger)

(i) Atropine – 0.25-1.0 mg orally, s/c, i/m or i/v
(ii) Hyoscine (Scopolamine) – 0.5 mg S/c
(iii) Hyoscyamine

(iv) Stramonium – 15-60 mg orally
(v) Tr. Belladona – 0.6 ml t.d.s.

B. Synthetic and Semisynthetic or Atropine substitutes

(i) *Acting on eye (Mydriatics)*
  — Homatropine hydrobromide sol – 2%
  — Dibutoline – 10-30 mg s/c
  — Cyclopentolate hydrochloride (Mydrilate) 0.5 – 1.0% sol
  — Eucatropine hydrochloride – 5-10% sol
  — Tropicamide (Mydriacyl)

(ii) *Spasmolytics (Antispasmodics)*
  — Homatropine methyl bromide ⎫
  — Oxyphenonium (Antrenyl) ⎬ 2-15 mg/day
  — Pipenzolate bromide (Piptal) ⎭
  — Propantheline (Probanthine) ⎫
  — Methantheline ⎪
  — Tricyclamol chloride ⎬ 50-100 mg/day
  — Adephenine ⎭
  — Dicyclimine hydrochloride ⎫
  — Oxyphencyclimine hydrochloride ⎬ 10 mg/day

(iii) *Anti-secretory drugs*
- Propantheline bromide (Probanthine)
- Oxyphenonium bromide (Antrenyl) ⎤
- Methantheline bromide (Banthine)   ⎬ Doses as described earlier
- Methscopolamine bromide (Pamine) ⎦

(iv) *Anti-parkinsonian drugs*
- Procyclidine (Kemadrine) – 2.5-40 mg/day orally
- Benztropine (Cogentin) – 0.5-6.0 mg/day orally
- Orphenadrine (Disipal) – 50-400 mg/day orally
- Cycrimine (Pagitane) – 2.5-20 mg/day orally
- Ethopropazine hydrochloride (Lysivane) – 50-500 mg/day orally
- Trihexyphenidyl (Artane) – 6-24 mg/day orally

5. Ganglion Blocking Agents

These drugs inhibit the passage of nerve impulse from preganglionic to postganglionic neurons. These are following:

A. *Classification depending upon chemical structure*
1. *Quaternary ammonium compounds*
   — Hexamethonium – 5-100 mg s/c or i/m
         2-50 mg I/V

- Tetraethylammonium (TEA)
- Pentamethonium – 2-50 mg I/V
- Bretylium tosylate
2. *Tertiary amines*
    - Pentolinium – 60-600 mg/day orally
        Or
        2-10 mg s/c.
3. *Secondary amines*
    - Pempidine – 10-100 mg/day orally
4. *Thiophanium compounds*
    - Trimetaphan (Arfonad) – By continuous or intermittent I/V infusion
    - Mecamylamine – 2.5-5.0 mg/t.d.s.

B. *Classification depending upon mode of action*
1. *Drugs acting by competitive antagonism*
    - Hexamethonium – 5-100 mg s/c or i/m
    - Tetraethyl, ammonium chloride (TEAC)

- Pentolinium
- Pentamethonium
- Mecamylamine
- Pempidine

2. *Non-competitive agents*
    (a) Drugs which mimic the action of acetylcholine without getting affected by cholinesterase
        - Nicotine
    (b) Drugs affecting the secretion of acetylcholine at ganglion synapse level.
        - Procaine (Local anaesthetic)
        - Botulinum toxin
    (c) Drugs preventing the synthesis of acetylcholine
        - Hemicholinium

CHAPTER II
CARDIOVASCULAR SYSTEM

1. ***Drugs influencing the cardiac rate***
   A. *Slowing of heart rate is by*
      (*i*) Drugs acting through medullary centre
         — Digitalis
         — Picrotoxin
         — Leptazol
         — Nikethamide
         — Morphine
         — Strophanthus
         — Squill
      (*ii*) Drugs acting on autonomic ganglia
         — Nicotine
         — Galsemum
         — Lobeline

- (iii) Drugs blocking Bundle of His
    - Digitalis
    - Strophanthus
    - Squill
- (iv) Drugs depressing ectopic focus of abnormal impulses
    - Quinidine
    - Procainamide

B. *Acceleration of heart rate is by*
- (i) Alcohol
    - Nitrites
- (ii) Drugs acting on autonomic ganglia
    - Nicotine
    - Lobeline
- (iii) Drugs acting on myocardium
    - Digitalis ⎤
    - Caffeine ⎬ In large doses
    - Strophanthin ⎦

(iv) Others
- Atropine group of drugs
- Adrenaline
- Isoprenaline
- Ephedrine

2. *Anti-arrhythmic drugs*

1. *Cardiac glycosides*

Cardiac glycoside	Dose of digitalisation I/V	Oral	Daily maintenance dose
Digoxin	0.75 – 1.5 mg	2 – 3 mg	0.25 – 0.75 mg
Digitoxin	1.0 – 1.2 mg	1 – 2 mg	0.05 – 0.3 mg
Lanatoside C	1.2 – 1.6 mg	6 mg	1.0 mg
Ouabin	0.25 – 0.5 mg	—	—

2. *Alkaloids*
   — Quinidine – 0.2 gm tab. administered 2 – 6 hourly (in gradually increasing dosages).
3. *Local anaesthetics*
   — Procainamide
   (a) In emergency – 100 mg I/V every five minutes maximum upto 1 gm.
   (b) For ventricular tachycardia – Initial dose 1 gm followed by 0.5 – 1.0 gm 4 hourly
   (c) For premature ventricular beats – 0.5 gm 4 – 6 hourly
      — Lidocaine – 1.2 mg/kg I/V- in 30 seconds as loading dose followed by 1 – 3 mg/mt as maintenance dose.
      — Procaine
4. *Adrenergic blocking agents*

β- receptor blockers — Propranolol – 40 – 120 mg/day orally
(Inderal) *Or*
1 – 10 mg I/V
— Pronethalol – 1 – 3 mg I/V

α-receptor blockers – Dibenamin
5. *Cholinergic drugs*
    — Methacholine
    — Edrophonium (Tensilon) – 10 mg I/V
    — Neostigmine – 0.2 – 2.0 mg s/c
6. *Cholinergic blockers*
    — Atropine – 0.5 – 1.0 mg I/V
7. *Antispasmodics*
    — Papaverine
    — Pethidine
8. *Antihistaminics*
    — Diphenhydramine
    — Antazoline
    — Mepyramine
    — Promethazine

9. *Antimalarial drugs*
   — Quinine
   — Chloroquine
   — Mepacraine
10. *Anti-epileptics*
    — Diphenylhydantoin sodium 250 mg slow I/V followed by 300 – 600 mg/day orally.
11. **Tranquillizers**
    — Hydroxyzine
    — Chlorpromazine
12. **Vasopressors (*sympathomimetics*)**
    — Metarminol (Aramine) – 2 – 10 mg I/V slowly
    — Isoprenaline
    — Adrenaline
    — Ephedrine

26 | *Classification of Drugs*

13. ***Miscellaneous***
    — Certain ions
        K^+
        Mg^+
        Ca^+
        Ba^+
    — Molar lactate
    — Corticosteroids
    — Electric shock therapy (7000 volts for 2 – 3 milli seconds).

3. ***Vasoconstrictors***
    A. Drugs acting on musculature of arterial wall
        — Vasopressin
        — Toxic doses of Digitalis
        — Barium

B. *Drugs acting via nervous mechanism*
   (a) Direct stimulation of vasomotor centre is done by
   — Nikethamide
   — Picrotoxine
   — Leptazol
   — Atropine
   — Digitalis
   — Cocaine
   — Caffein
   — Camphor
   — CO_2 inhalation
   (b) Reflex stimulation of vasomotor centre is done by
   — Nikethamide
   — CO_2
   — Counter irritants

(c) By stimulation of sympathetic ganglion cells
- Nicotine
- Lobeline

(d) Sympathomimetic drugs
- Adrenaline
- Nor-drin
- Ephedrine
- Amphetamine
- Methamphetamine
- Nephazoline
- Phenylephrine

4. Vasodilators

These drugs dilate the arterioles and capillaries either directly or through vasomotor nerve.

1. *Drugs acting directly on vessels*
   - Organic nitrites and nitrates

- Xanthines
  - Aminophylline
  - Theophylline
- Nicotinic acid
- Papaverine
- Isoxsuprine
- Cyclandelate
- Histamine

2. **Adrenergic blocking agents**
   — Phentolamine (Regitine) – 5 – 30 mg I/M or I/V
   — Tolazoline (Priscol) – 25 – 50 mg orally, I/M or I/V 6 hourly
   — Dibenamine – 4 – 6 mg/kg body weight, Maximum single dose 100 mg
   — Propranolol – 10 – 40 mg orally 6 – 8 hourly, I/V slowly.

3. **Parasympathomimetics**
   — Methacholine

- Carbachol – 0.2 – 0.5 mg/S/C or 1 – 4 mg orally
- Pilocarpine
- Physostigmine

4. **Ganglion blockers**
   - Pempidine
   - Mecamylamine
   - Methonium compounds

5. **Drugs acting on higher centres**
   - Reserpine
   - Apresoline

6. **Drugs acting on vasomotor centre**
   - Narcotics
   - Reserpine
   - General anaesthetics
   - Alcohol

5. Hypotensive or Antihypertensive drugs

Drugs which lower the blood pressure are known as hypotensive agents.

These are:
1. *Drugs acting on higher centres (in brain)*
   — Rauwolfia alkaloids (Reserpine) – 0.3 – 1.0 mg daily orally or I/M
   — Hydralazine (Apresoline) – 100 – 500 mg/day orally
   — Sedatives
   — Hypnotics viz Phenobarbitone
   — Tranquillizers — Meprobamate
                      — Chlorpromazine
2. *Drugs acting on vasomotor centre in medulla oblongata*
   — Ergot alkaloids viz Hydergin – 0.3 mg/day
   — Morphine.

3. *Ganglion blocking agents*
   — Pempidine bitartrate (Perolysen) – 10 – 100 mg/day orally
   — Hexamethonium – 5 – 100 mg I/M
   — Mecamylamine hydrochloride – 10 – 120 mg/day orally
   — Pentolinium – 60 – 1500 mg/day orally
   — T.E.A
4. *Adrenergic blocking agents*
   — Tolazoline
   — Piperoxan
   — Guanethidine (Ismelin) 10 – 200 mg/day orally
   — Methyl dopa (Aldomet) – 0.5 – 2.5 gm/day
   — Bretylium – 300 mg – 3.00 gm/day orally
   — Bethanidine – 20 – 200 mg/day orally
   — Guanoxan – 120 mg/day

5. *Drugs acting on blood vessels (smooth musculature of blood vessels)*
   — Methyl dopa
   — Hydralazine
   — Sodium nitrite
   — Mannitol hexanitrate
   — Aminophylline
   — Sodium nitroprusside
6. *Diuretics (By reducing plasma volume)*
   — Thiazides
   — Spironolactones
   — Fursemide
7. *Drugs blocking renin angiotensin system*
   — Betablockers
   — Saralasin

6. Coronary Dilators
Or
Anti Anginal Drugs

1. *Nitrites and Nitrates (Drugs acting directly on coronary vessels)*

	Initial oral dose	Initial sublingual dose
— Nitroglycerine	—	0.5 – 6.0 mg/day (with individual variation)
— Sorbitrate (Isosorbide Dinitrate)	10 mg	5 mg
— Peritrate	20 – 60 mg t.d.s. orally or s/l	—
— Mannitol hexanitrate	15 – 60 mg orally	—
— Erythrityl tetranitrate	7.5 – 15 mg s/l	—

2. *Synthetic drugs*
   — Isoptin (verapamil) – 120 – 240 mg orally/day

- Segontin (Prenylamine) – 120 – 240 mg/day orally
- Persantin (Dipyramidol) – 75 –150 mg/day orally

3. *Adrenergic drugs*
   - Adrenaline ⎤
   - Nor-adrenaline ⎬ Not used clinically
   - Ephedrine ⎦
4. *β-adrenergic blocking agents*
   - Propranolol – 10 – 30 mg t.d.s. orally
   - Sotalol
5. *M. A. O. inhibitors*
   - Phenelazine
   - Iproniazide
6. *Alkaloids*
   - Khelline
7. *Miscellaneous*
   - Nicotinic acid
   - Antithyroid drugs
   - Anticoagulants

7. Drugs used in peripheral vascular diseases

- Tolazoline – 75 – 150 mg/day orally
- Phentolamine – 5 – 10 mg I/M or I/V
- Isoxsuprine – 6 – 30 mg/day orally
- Dibenzyline
- Nylidrine – 10 –40 mg/day orally
- Alcohol
- Methonium compounds
- Histamine
- Glycine
- Complamina (Xanthinol nicotinate – 300 mg/day orally)
- Nicotinic acid – 100 – 500 mg/day orally

8. Drugs used in Atherosclerosis

1. *Drugs decreasing the uptake of cholesterol from G. I. T.*
   - Sitosterol
   - Neomycin

2. *Drugs which decrease the release of cholesterol from adipose tissues*
   — Nicotinic acid
3. *Drugs inhibiting the synthesis of cholesterol*
   — Triparanol
   — Nicotinic acid
   — Clofibrate
4. *Drugs which increase cholesterol catabolism*
   — Dextrothyroxine
5. *Drugs increasing removal of cholesterol*
   — Heparine.

CHAPTER III
RESPIRATORY SYSTEM

1. Bronchodilators or Bronchial Antispasmodics

1. *Sympathomimetics*
   — Adrenaline 0.1 – 0.5 ml (1 : 1000) S/C
   — Ephedrine 30 – 60 mg t.d.s. or 1 – 1.5% nasal drops
   — Isoprenaline 10-20 mg sublingually s.o.s.
   — Orcipre naline – 20 mg 6 hourly orally
2. *Parasympathomimetic blocking agents*
   — Atropine
   — Hyoscine or Tincture hyoscyamus
   — Stramonium
3. *Ganglion blocking agents*
   — Large doses of Lobelia
4. *C. N. S. depressants*
   — Sedatives and Hypnotics

5. *Drugs acting directly on bronchial muscles*
   — Xanthine derivatives viz Aminophylline 250 mg I/V slowly
   — Theophylline
   — Papaverine
   — Nitrites
6. *Miscellaneous*
   — Cortisone-gradually increasing/tapering dosages
   — ACTH
   — Anti-histaminics
   — Terbutaline aerosols
   — Potassium iodide

2. Respiratory Stimulants

1. *Direct stimulants of Respiratory centre*
   (a) Alkaloids
      — Atropine
      — Caffeine 0.2 – 0.3 gm
      — Strychnine

- Lobelline
- Picrotoxin
  (b) Synthetic drugs
  - Nikethamide
  - Amphetamine
  - Leptazol
2. *Reflex stimulants*
   - CO_2 – 5 – 7%
   - Ammonia inhalation
   - Aromatic spirit of ammonia
   - Oxygen insufficiency
   - Mustard bath
   - Camphor
3. *Drugs acting by competitive antagonism*
   - Nalorphine (in morphine poisoning) 5 – 10 mg I/V
   - Daptazole (in poisoning by morphine and narcotic analgesic

— Bemegride (in Barbiturate poisoning) 500 mg in 100 mg of Normal saline I/V

3. Respiratory Depressants

A. *Drugs acting directly on Respiratory centre*

1. *Narcotic analgesics*
   — Morphine 10 – 15 mg I/M
   — Pethidine 100 mg I/M
   — Methadone 5 – 10 mg 4 hourly S/C or orally
   — Opium

2. *Hypnotics*
   — Barbiturates – Dosage depends on individual product
   — Large doses of alcohol
   — Chloral hydrate 0.6 gm.

3. *General anaesthetics*
   — Chloroform
   — Ether
   — Nitrous oxide
   — Cyclopropane

4. *Miscellaneous*
   — Aconite
   — Hydrocyanic acid

B. ***Drugs acting reflexly on respiratory centre***
   — CO_2 insufficiency

4. Antitussive (Cough sedatives)
Or
Cough Suppressants

A. ***Centrally acting— (These depress the cough centre in brainstem)***
   1. *Addictive*
      — Morphine – 10 – 15 mg S/C or I/M
      — Heroin (Dimorphine) – 5 – 10 mg orally or 3 –6 mg S/C
      — Methadione – 5 – 10 mg 4 hourly orally or S/C
      — Camphorated tincture of opium

2. *Non-addictive*
    — Codeine – 10 – 60 mg
    — Pholcodeine – 5 –15 mg
    — Noscapine – 15 – 50 mg
    — Pipezethate (Selvigon)
    — Dextromethorphan (Romilar) 15 – 30 mg orally
3. *Antihistaminics*
    — Diphenhydramine – 25 – 50 mg orally
    — Chlorphenaramine – 8 –12 mg capsules
    — Promethazine – 25 –75 mg orally

B. *Peripherally acting*
1. *Drugs liquefying tenacious bronchial secretions*
   Expectorants
    — Ipecacuanha
    — Ammonium chloride

44 | *Classification of Drugs*

- Creosote
- Potassium iodide

2. *Mucolytic agents*
   - CO_2 inhalation
   - Steam inhalation

3. *Drugs depressing the sensory receptors in upper respiratory tract*
   - Tincture Benzoin inhalation
   - Cocaine inhalation
   - Demulscents
   - Menthol spray

5. Expectorants

Stimulant expectorants (Mainly aromatic expectorants)
   Volatile oils
   - Camphor
   - Creosote

- Terpine hydrate
- Guaiacol

Sedative expectorants

1. *Saline expectorants.* They liquefy the tenacious sputum, increase bronchial secretions and stimulate effective cough.

   Used in mixtures
   - Potassium iodide – 250 – 500 mg
   - Ammonium chloride – 300 – 400 mg
   - Ammonium bicarbonate 300 – 600 mg
   - Sodium citrate
   - Potassium citrate

2. *Nauseating expectorants*
   - Ipecacuanah
   - Scilla
   - Apomorphine – 2 – 8 mg S/C

3. *Demulscent expectorants*
   - Liquorice
   - Gum acacia

- Syrups
- Glycerine
4. *Anodyne expectorants* – They depress the cough reflex. These are opium and its alkaloids viz.
   - Morphine – 10 –15 mg I/M
   - Codeine – 8 – 15 mg in elixir form
   - Pholcodeine – 5 – 15 mg orally
   - Norcapine – 15 – 30 mg.

CHAPTER IV
DRUGS ACTING ON GASTROINTESTINAL TRACT

1. Bitters

These are the drugs that stimulate appetite and digestion by increasing gastric secretions.

Classification

1. *Simple bitters*
    — Quassia
    — Columba
    — Chirata
2. *Aromatic bitters*
    — Tr. lemon or lemon peel
    — Tr. orange or bitter orange peel
3. *Alkaloid bitters*
    — Quinine
    — Strychnine

4. *Astringent bitters*
   — Tannic acid
   — Kalmegh

2. Carminatives

These are the drugs that relieve flatulence. These are:
   — Tr. card co
   — Tr. gengibaris
   — Camphor
   — Anise
   — Peppermint
   — Coriander
   — Cinnamon

3. Gastric Antacids

These are the drugs which are used to diminish Hydrochloric acid in stomach.

1. *Systemic antacids*
   — Sodium bicarbonate – (1.5 gm)

Drugs Acting on Gastrointestinal Tract | **49**

- — Sodium citrate
- — Sodium acetate
2. *Non-systemic antacids*
    - — Aluminium compounds viz. Al. hydroxide gel – 15 – 30 ml
    - — Aluminium phosphate – 4 – 8 ml
    - — Dihydroxy Al. amino acetate
    - — Gastric mucin – 2 – 5 gm
    - — Magnesium oxide – 0.25 gm – 0.5 gm
    - — Magnesium trisilicate – 1 gm
    - — Calcium carbonate – 1.5 gm
    - — Magnesia magma
    - — Ion exchange resins – 0.5 – 1 gm
    - — Milk

4. Digestants

These are the drugs which are used to replace certain elements natural digestive processes which are lacking in body.

- Dilute hydrochloric acid
- Glutamic acid
- Betanine hydrochloride
- Renin
- Pepsin
- Pancreatin
- Bile salts

5. Emetics

The drugs which induce vomiting are known as emetics.

1. *Reflex (Local) Emetics*
   - Sodium chloride (Hypertonic solution)
   - Mustard
   - Zinc sulfate
   - Copper sulfate
   - Antimony tartarate
   - Ipecacuanha

2. *Central or Direct Emetics*
   — Apomorphine hydrochloride
3. *Drugs inducing vomiting*
   — Digitalis
   — Salicylates
   — Morphine
   — Picrotoxin
   — Emetine
   — Veratrum alkaloids

6. Antiemetics

The drugs which are used to check vomiting are known as antiemetics

1. ***Centrally acting antiemetics***
   (*a*) Tranquillisers (Phenothiazine derivatives)
      — Chlorpromazine (Largetil – 25 – 50 mg t.d.s.

- Triflupromazine (Siquil) – 10 – 25 mg b.d. orally
- Trifluoperazine (Eskazine) – 2–5 mg 8 hourly
- Prochlorperazine (Stemetil) – 15 – 30 mg orally daily

(b) Antihistaminics
- Diphenhydramine – 25 – 50 mg b.d.
- Dramamine – 100 mg t.d.s.
- Trimeton – 25 mg b.d.
- Avomine – 25 mg b.d.
- Promethazine – 25 mg b.d.
- Pheneramine maleate – 40 mg b.d.

(c) Vitamins
- Pyridoxin (Vit. B_6)

(d) Hypnotics
- Barbiturates
- Bromides

- Chloral hydrate – 0.6 gm
- Hyoscine

2. *Locally acting antiemetics*

   (a) Those forming protective layer over gastric mucosa
   - Calcium carbonate
   - Bismuth carbonate
   - Kaolin

   (b) Those producing sedative action on gastric mucosa
   - Cocaine
   - Menthol
   - Sodium bicarbonate
   - Chlorbutol

   (c) Miscellaneous
   - Mustard plaster (Counter irritant)
   - Sucking ice cubes

7. Intestinal Spasmodics

These are the drugs which produce muscular spasm of intestinal musculature.

1. *Acting through nervous mechanism (Parasympathomimetic drugs)*
   — Methacholine – 10 – 40 mg S/C
   — Carbachol – 2 mg orally, 0.25 mg S/C, 1.5% sol. locally.
   — Physostigmine – 0.5% sol. locally
   — Pilocarpine – 0.5 – 4% locally (Nitrate or Hydrochloride salt)

2. *Drugs acting directly on intestinal muscles*
   — Histamine
   — Vasopressin
   — Salts of lead, barium and calcium

8. Intestinal Antispasmodics

These drugs release the muscular spasm of intestinal tract.

1. *Sympathomimetic drugs*
    — Adrenaline
    — Ephedrine
    — Amphetamine
2. *Parasympatholytic drugs*
    — Atropine – 0.6 mg
    — Hyoscine
    — Belladona
    — Probanthin – 15 mg b.d.
    — Oxyphenonium bromide (Antrenyl) – 5-10 mg q.i.d.
3. *Drugs acting directly on intestinal musculature*
    — Nitrites
    — Papaverine
    — Potassium salts
    — Pethidine

9. Purgatives

These are the drugs which promote peristalsis and evacuation of intestinal contents (defecation).

A. *Irritant purgatives*
1. *Emodine purgatives*
   — Cascara sagrada – 2-4 ml
   — Aloes – 2-5 gr
   — Senna – 5-20 gr
   — Rhuarb – 3-15 gr
2. *Resinous purgatives or cathartics*
   — Jalap
   — Colocynt
   — Podophyllum
   — Elaterin
3. *Irritant oils*
   — Castor oil – 15 ml
   — Croton oil – 0.6 ml

4. *Miscellaneous*
   — Phenolphthalein 60-300 mg
   — Calomel – 30-120 mg
   — Liquorice
   — Bisacodyl – 2 tabs of 5 mg each s.o.s.

B. Bulk forming cathartics or purgatives
   1. *Saline purgatives*

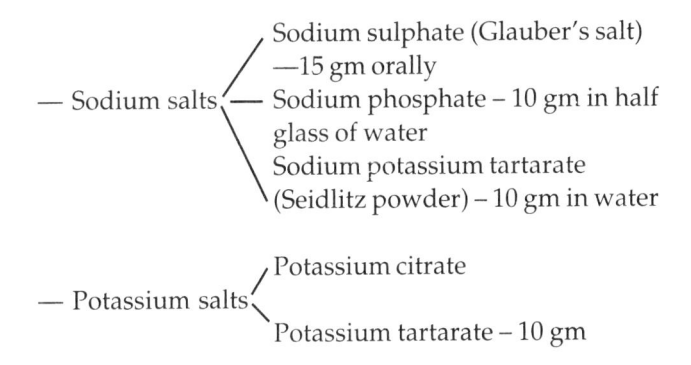

   — Sodium salts
   - Sodium sulphate (Glauber's salt) —15 gm orally
   - Sodium phosphate – 10 gm in half glass of water
   - Sodium potassium tartarate (Seidlitz powder) – 10 gm in water

   — Potassium salts
   - Potassium citrate
   - Potassium tartarate – 10 gm

- Magnesium salts
  - Magnesium sulfate (Epsom salt) – 15 gm orally
  - Magnesia magma (Milk of magnesia) – 15 ml
  - Magnesium carbonate

2. *Colloidal purgatives*
   - Bran
   - Isaphgol
   - Agar
   - Methyl cellulose – 1-4 gm powder orally
   - Tragacanth
   - Gum acacia

C. ***Emollient cathartics***
   - Liquid paraffin
   - Vegetable oils
     - Olive oil,
     - Cotton seed oil

Drugs Acting on Gastrointestinal Tract | **59**

D. *Miscellaneous*

Parasympathomimetic and other drugs
— Acetylcholine injection
— Physostigmine
— Carbachol
— Pilocarpine
— Post-pituitary extract

10. Intestinal Astringents

These are the drugs which bind or arrest the secretions in intestinal tract.

1. Mineral or metallic astringents
   Salts of:—
   — Lead

- Zinc
- Aluminium
- Silver
- Copper

2. *Vegetable astringents*
   - Catechu (Katha)
   - Krameria (root)
   - Hamamelis (Leaves)
   - Activated charcol.

CHAPTER V
CENTRAL NERVOUS SYSTEM

Classification of drugs acting on C.N.S.

1. Hypnotics
2. Analgesics
3. General anaesthetics
4. Antiepileptics
5. Pyretics
6. Antipyretics
7. C.N.S. stimulants
8. Tranquilizers
9. Anti-depressants
10. Psychotogenic drugs

1. Hypnotics

There are the drugs which induce sleep closely resembling the natural sleep.

I. *Barbiturate hypnotics*

(a) *Long acting barbiturates (Action lasts 8-12 hours)*
— Phenobarbitone (Luminal, Gardinal) – 80-120 mg/orally/day or I/M

- Barbitone (Barbital, Medinal)
- Methylphenobarbitone (Prominal, Phemitone) 60—200 mg orally

(b) *Intermediate acting barbiturates* (*Action lasts 4-8 hours*)
- Amylobarbitone (Amytal) – 0.1-0.2 gm orally
- Butobarbitone (Soneryl) – 0.1-0.2 gm orally
- Allobarbitone – 30-200 mg orally
- Vinbarbitone – 30-200 mg orally

(c) *Short acting barbiturates*
- Pentobarbitone (Nembutal) – 100-300 mg orally
- Secobarbitone (Seconal) – 100-200 mg orally
- Hepatobarbitone – 200-400 mg
- Cyclobarbitone – 200-400 mg orally

(d) *Ultra short acting barbiturates*
- Hexobarbitone sodium (Evapan) – 200-400 mg I/V
- Surital – 0.2-1.0 gm I/V

II. Non-barbiturate hypnotics

(a) *Chloral derivatives*
— Chloral hydrate
  - As sedative — 0.25 gm orally
  - As hypnotic — 0.5–1.0 gm orally
  - Rectal dose — 0.5–1.0 gm
— Chloral formamide
— Butyl chloral hydrate
— Chlorobutanol – 600 mg orally

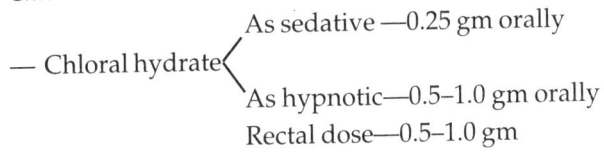

(b) *Aldehyde group*
— Paraldehyde – 5-10 ml orally, Deep I/M or rectally

(c) *Bromides*
— Potassium bromide – 300 mg - 1.5 gm orally
— Sodium bromide – 300 mg - 1.5 gm orally
— Ammonium bromide – 300 mg – 1.5 gm orally

64 | *Classification of Drugs*

- (d) *Urea derivatives*
  - Carbromal (Adalin) – 300 mg – 1.000 gm orally
  - Bromvaletone – 300-600 mg orally
  - Ectyl urea – 150-300 mg orally
- (e) *Piperidine derivatives*
  - Glutethimide (Doriden) – 250-500 mg orally
  - Methyprylon (Noludar) 200-400 mg orally
- (f) *Carbonic acid esters of glycol alcohol*
  - Meprobamate (Equanil or Miltown) – 20-40 mg/kg/day
  - Ethinamate (Valmid) – 500 mg – 1.000 gm
  - Urethane
  - Placidyl – 500 mg
- (g) *Benzodiazepine derivatives*
  - Chlordiazepoxide (Librium) – 10-40 mg orally
  - Diazepam (Calmpose) – 5-15 mg orally
  - Oxazepam (Serepex) – 15-45 mg orally
- (h) *Alcohols*
  - Amylene hydrate
  - Bromethol

- Ethyl alcohol
- Tribromoethanol

(i) *Miscellaneous*
— Antihistaminics
  — Diphenhydramine – 25-50 mg b.d.
  — Pyrilamine – 25-50 mg b.d.
  — Hydroxyzine – 25 mg t.d.s
— Parasympatholytics
  — Hyoscine
  — Magnesium sulfate when used I/V

2. **Analgesics**

These are the drugs which relieve pain

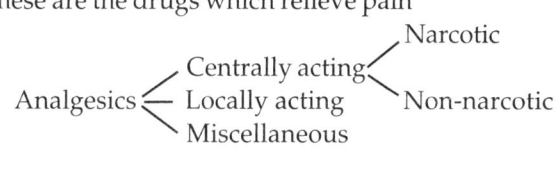

```
                          ╱ Narcotic
            Centrally acting
Analgesics ← Locally acting
            ╲ Miscellaneous  ╲ Non-narcotic
```

Centrally Acting Analgesics

Narcotic analgesics —These act on cerebral cortex and thalamus

— Opium
— Morphine – 10-15 mg I/M, S/C, I/V
— Codeine – 10-60 mg orally
— Heroin – 4-8 mg
— Ethylmorphine (Dionin) – 2-5% aqueous sol
— Pethidine – 50-150 mg I/M
— Dilaudid – 3 mg I/M
— Metopon – 5 mg orally
— Oxymorphone
— Methadone – 5 mg 4 hourly, 10 mg S/C for excruciating pain

Non-narcotic Analgesics (Acting on thalamus)
A. *Anti-pyretic analgesics* (Coal-tar derivatives)
   — Sodium salicylate – 0.6-2.0 gm/day orally, high dosages in rheumatism
   — Acetyl salicylic acid – 0.3-1.0 gm/day (Aspirin), high dosages in rheumatism
   — Salicylamide
   — Methyl salicylate (Oil of Wintergreen)
B. *Paraminophenol derivatives*
   — Acetanilid – 0.12-0.30 gm orally
   — Phenacetin – 300-600 mg orally
   — Paracetamol – 0.5-1.000 gm orally
C. *Pyrazolon derivatives*
   — Amidopyrin – 300-600 mg/day
   — Antipyrine
   — Phenylbutazone – 300-600 mg/day

D. *Propionic acid derivatives*
- Ibuprofen – 200-400 mg/orally
- Ketoprofen – 150 mg/day orally
- Oxyphenbutazone – 100-400 mg/day

E. *Miscellaneous*
- Metamizole (Analgin) – 250 mg – 1.000 gm orally or I/M
- Indomethacin (Indocid) – 50-150 mg/day orally

Locally acting analgesics

Drugs acting on nerve trunks
- Local anaesthetics
- Alcohol infiltrated locally

Drugs acting on end organs (i.e. Skin)

(*a*) Heat

(*b*) Cold
- Physical e.g. ice
- Chemical e.g. Ethyl chloride

(c) Chemicals
- Mustard oil
- Methyl salicylate
- Clove oil
- Turpentine

Local anodynes
— Belladonna plaster
— Volatile oils
— Phenols
— Chloretone

Miscellaneous
— Procain and procainamide
— Spasmolytics – in colics
— Colchicine – in gout
— Steroids and ACTH – in Rheumatism
— Nitrites – In angina pectoris

3. **General Anaesthetics**

The drugs which abolish the perception of stimuli, obliterate motor activity and produce a hiatus in consciousness are known as general anaesthetics.

- (a) Volatile anaesthetics
- (b) Non-volatile anaesthetics

(a) *Volatile anaesthetics*

(1) *Liquids*
- Ether – 5-10% in inspired air
- Chloroform – 0.5-1.5% in inspired air
- Vinyl ether
- Halothane – 1-4% in inspired air
- Trilene
- Ethyl chloride

(2) *Gases*
- Nitrous oxide – 65% + 35% O_2
- Ethylene – 80-90% with O_2
- Cyclopropane – 15-20% with O_2

(b) *Non-volatile general anaesthetics*
- Thiopentone sodium
- Paraldehyde
- Suritol sodium
- Hydroxydione sodium succinate
- Ketalor – 4-6 mg/kg I/M or 1-2 mg/kg I/V

4. **Anti-epileptic Drugs**

   These are the drugs which control epileptic seizures.

   A. *Classification according to chemical structure*:

   I. *Bromides:* Pot. Bromide 0.3-1.2 gm (O)

   II. *Barbiturates:*
   1. Phenobarbitone – 60-300 mg/day orally or I/M
   2. Mephobarbitone – 60-200 mg orally
   3. Methabarbitone – 100-600 mg/day orally

III. *Hydantoins:*
  1. Diphenyl hydantoin (Dilantin, phenytoin) – 300-600 mg/day orally
  2. Ethotoin (Peganone) – 2-3 gm/day orally
  3. Mephenytoin (Mesantoin) – 300-600 gm/day orally

IV. *Pyrimidine derivatives:*
  — Primidone (Mysolin) – 250 mg – 2.0 mg/day orally

V. *Oxazolidinediones:*
  1. Trimethadione (Tridone) – 600-1200 mg/day orally
  2. Paramethadione (Paradione) – 0.6-1.8 gm/day orally

VI. *Succinimides:*
  1. Ethosuximide (Zarontin) – 500-1500 mg/day orally
  2. Methsuximide (Celontin) – 600-1200 mg/day orally
  3. Phensuximide (Milontin) – 0.5-4 gm/day orally

VII. *Phenylacetylureas*
  1. Phenacemide – 1.5-5 gm/day orally
  2. Pheneturide – 0.2-1 gm/day orally

VIII. *Benzodiazepines:*
   1. Nitrazepam – 5-10 mg orally
   2. Diazepam – 10-30 mg/day orally

IX. *Amides*
   1. Aminoglutethimide
   2. Atrolactamide

X. *Miscellaneous*
   1. Carbamazepine (Mezetol) – 0.3-1.2 gm/day orally
   2. Paraldehyde – 4-8 ml I/M
   3. Acetazolamide (Diamox) – 250-1000 mg/day orally
   4. Chlordiazepoxide
   5. Meprobamate – 1.2-2 gm/day
   6. Methyl parafynol
   7. Sodium valproate – 600-1600 mg/day

B. Classification according to clinical uses

I. Drugs used in Grand mal and Jacksonian epilepsy (Major epilepsy)

(a) 1. *Cortical depressants* (*Barbiturates*)
   — Phenobarbitone 100-300 mg/day
   — Methabarbitone

2. *Hydantoins*
   — Dilantin sodium – 3-8 mg/kg/day
   — Mesentoin 300-600 mg/day
   — Ethotoin 2-3 gm/day

3. *Pyrimidine derivatives*
   — Mysoline – 250 mg - 2 gm/day

4. *Bromides*
   — Sodium bromide
   — Ammonium bromide
   — Potassium bromide

II. Drugs used in Petit mal epilepsy

1. *Succinimide derivatives*
   — Ethsuximide (Zarontin) – 20-30 mg/kg/day
   — Methsuximide (Celontin) – 15-20 mg/kg/day
   — Phenusuccimide (Melontin) – 20-40 mg/kg/day
2. *Oxazolidine derivatives*
   — Trimethadione – 20-50 mg/kg/day
   — Paradione
   — Malidine
3. *Diuretics*
   — Acetazolamide – 15-30 mg/kg/day

III. Drugs used in Psychomotor epilepsy

— Pyrimidine derivatives e.g. Mysoline – 12-25 mg/kg/day
— Hydantoins e.g. Dilantin sodium – 3-8 mg/kg/day
— Phenyl acetyl urea
— Mezetol

IV *Drugs used in Status epilepticus*
— Pentothal sodium
— Barbiturates
— Hydantoins
— Diazepam
— Paraldehyde
— General anaesthetics

5. Pyretics

A. *Physical methods*

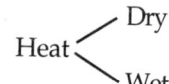

Heat — Dry
Heat — Wet

B. *By injecting foreign proteins*
— Various vaccinations
— Milk protein

C. *Drugs*
— Picrotoxin
— Cocaine

D. *Malarial fever therapy*
- By injecting 5 c.c defibrinated blood containing benign tertiary malarial parasite.

6. Anti-pyretics

Drugs which lower the body temperature are known as anti-pyretics

Non-specific Anti-pyretics

(i) *Physical agents: Local applications viz.*
- Cold sponging
- Ice cap
- Using evaporating substances, viz. Surface anaesthetics

(ii) *Diaphoretics*
- Sodium citrate
- Potassium citrate
- Alcohol
- Pilocarpine

- Opium
- Liq. ammon. Acetate

(*iii*) *Analgesics*
- Sodium salicylate – 0.6-2.0 gm, orally
- Aspirin – 0.6 gm – 1.0 gm, orally
- Aminopyrin – 0.3 gm
- Paracetamol – 500 mg
- Acetanilid – 0.2 gm

Specific anti-pyretics – These drugs lower the body temperature by attacking the cause of fever.

For infection – specific and suitable antibiotics, sulfa drugs, etc.

For malaria – anti-malarials

For tuberculosis – anti-T.B. drugs

7. **CNS Stimulants**

   These drugs act at various sites in CNS

   I. *Drugs acting on cerebral cortex*

   A. Xanthines
   — Caffein – 200 mg. – 400 mg, orally

- B. *Sympathomimetics*
  - Methedrine – 2.5-5.0 mg orally
  - Dexedrine – 15-20 mg daily in divided dosages
  - Amphetamine – 5-10 mg orally or S/C
  - Ephedrine – 30-60 mg t.d.s.
- C. *Parasympatholytics*
  - Atropine – 0.6 mg
- D. *Local anaesthetics*
  - Cocaine
- E. *Anti-depressants*
  - Impiramine (Depsonil) – 50-500 mg daily

II. **Medullary stimulants**
  - Leptazol – 0.5-1.0 ml 10% sol. I/V
  - Picrotoxin
  - Bemegride – 500 mg in 100 ml of N. Saline I/V

80 | Classification of Drugs

- Nikethamide – 1.5-3.0 ml I/M or I/V ⎫
- Nicotine ⎪ Indirect
- Ammonium carbonate inhalation ⎬ and Reflex
- Spirit ammonium aromaticus orally ⎭ Stimulants

III. *Spinal cord stimulants*
- Strychnine hydrochloride – 2-8 mg orally
- Thebaine

8. Tranquilizers (Psycholeptics)

A. *Major tranquilizers*

1. *Phenothiazine derivatives*
    - Chlorpromazine (Largactil) 25-100 mg q.i.d.
    - Promazine (Sparine) 25-300 mg t.d.s.
    - Triflupromazine (Siquil) 25-75 mg t.d.s.
    - Trifluperazine (Eskazine) 1-8 mg t.d.s
    - Prochlorperazine (Stemetil) 5-15 mg t.d.s.
    - Trimeprazine (Vallergan)

2. *Rauwolfia alkaloids*
    — Reserpine (Serpasil) 0.5-2.5 mg b.d.
    — Deserpidine 2-3 mg/day
    — Methoserpidine

B. *Intermediate tranquilizers*
    — Haloperidol (Serenace)
    — Trifluperidol

C. *Minor tranquilizers*
    — Promethazine (Phenergan) – 12.5 mg b.d.
    — Hydroxyzine (Atarax) 75-100 mg daily

D. *Miscellaneous*
    — Meprobamate (Equanil) 600-1200 mg/daily
    — Chlordiazepoxide (Librium) 10-40 mg/daily
    — Diazepam (Calmpose) 15-40 mg/daily
    — Oxazepam (Serepax) 15-45 mg/daily

9. Anti-depressants

These drugs are also known as Thymoleptics or psychoanaleptics and are used to remove depression.

M.A.O. (Monoamine oxidase) inhibitors

— Marsilid – not used clinically because of its toxic effects
— Nialamide (Niamid) – 75 mg daily
— Marplan – 30 mg daily
— Nardil – 15 mg t.d.s.

Sympathomimetics

— Amphetamine – 5-10 mg orally or S/C
— Methamphetamine 2.5-5 mg orally t.d.s.
— Dexamphetamine – 15-20 mg daily in divided doses

Miscellaneous

— Methyl tryptamine
— Cocaine

Iminodibenzyl derivatives
- Impiramine (Dapsonil) – 100-300 mg daily
- Amitriptyline – 75-150 mg daily in divided doses
- Orphenadrine

Piperidine derivatives
- Ritalin 5-10 mg t.d.s.
- Meratran 2-6 mg daily

10. Psychotogenic drugs (Hallucinogens)

These drugs create a state of mental confusion and are used only in experimental animals for study purposes.

- L.S.D. 25
- Adrenochrome
- Mescaline
- Marihuana
- Phencyclidine

CHAPTER VI
DRUGS ACTING ON URINARY SYSTEM

1. **Diuretics**
   Substances which increase the urinary output are known as diuretics.

   Classification
   1. *Water* (Physiological diuretic)
   2. *Alkalies* — Pot. Citrate, Pot. Bicarbonate, Pot. Acetate, Sod. Citrate, Sod. Bicarbonate, Sod. Acetate
   3. *Acid* – Ammon. Chloride, Cal. Chloride, Mandalic acid
   4. *Benzothiadiazine derivatives*
      — Chlorthiazide – 0.5-2.0 gm daily
      — Hydrochlorthiazide (Esidrix) – 25-100 mg daily
      — Cyclothiazide – 2-8 mg daily
      — Polythiazide (Nephril) 1.4 mg daily
      — Frusemide (Lasix) – (40-120 mg/day orally or 20-40 mg I/V or I/M)
      — Cyclopenthiazide – 1-2 mg orally

5. *Mercurials*
    - Mersalyl – 200 mg/day
    - Meralluride 0.5-2.0 ml I/M or S/C
    - Mercaptomerine – 0.5-2.0 ml S/C on alternate day or twice a week
    - Mercuderamde – 0.5-2.0 ml I/M twice or thrice a week
6. *Xanthines*
    - Caffeine – 250-500 mg orally
    - Theophylline – 60-200 mg orally
    - Aminophylline – 100-300 mg orally or 250-500 mg I/V slowly
7. *Carbonic anhydrase inhibitors*
    - Acetazolamide (Diamox) – 500 mg/day orally
    - Methazolamide – 50-100 mg orally b.d./t.d.s.
    - Ethoxzolamide – 125-250 mg daily
    - Dichlorphenamide – 50-100 mg orally

8. *Aminouracil derivatives*
   — Chlorthalidone (Hygrotone) 50-100 mg/day
   — Triamterene 50-200 mg/day
   — Aminometradine (Mictine) 200-800 mg/day
9. *Aldosterone antagonists*
   — Spironolactone 100-200 mg daily
10. *Osmotic diuretics*
    Electrolytes
    — Sodium chloride
    — Sodium sulfate
    — Potassium chloride
    — Potassium nitrate
    Non-electrolytes
    — Glucose
    — Sorbitol
    — Mannitol
    — Sucrose
    — Urea

Substances increasing colloidal osmotic pressure
- Dextran
- PVP
- Albumin
- Acacia

11. *Miscellaneous*
    - Ethcrynic acid 50-200 mg/day

2. Urinary Antiseptics

1. *Alkalies* (Urinary alkalizers)
   - Sodium and potassium bicarbonate
   - Sodium and potassium citrate
   - Sodium and potassium acetate

2. *Acids* (Urinary acidifiers)
   - Ammonium chloride – 3-6 gm/day orally
   - Sodium acid phosphate
   - Mandelic acid

3. *Sulpha drugs*

	Initial dose	Subsequent dose
— Sulfadimidine		
— Sulfadiazine	4-6 gm	1-1.5 gm hrly
— Sulfasomidine	1 gm 8 hrly	
— Sulfamethiazol	0.5 gm 4 hrly	

4. *Antibiotics*
   - Tetracycline   250 mg 6 hrly
   - Ampicillin – 500 mg I/M or I/V 6 hrly
   - Kanamycin – 15 mg/kg daily in divided doses
   - Chloramphenicol – 250-500 mg 6 hrly
   - Cycloserine – 0.5 gm orally daily
   - Polymyxin B – 2.5 mg/kg/day I/M
   - Colomycin 2.5-5.0 mg/kg/day I/M

5. *Nitrofurantoin derivatives*
   - Nitrofurantoin (Furadantin) – 5-8 mg/kg body weight daily

6. *Salts of organic acids*
   — Calcium mandelate
   — Ammonium mandelate
   — Methenamine mandelate (Mandalamine) – 4 gm/day
7. *Naphthyridine derivatives*
   — Nalidixic acid (Gramoneg) 3-4 gm/day
8. *Dyes*
   — Pyridium 200 mg t.d.s. orally
   — Hexyl resorcinol
   — Acriflavin
9. *Essential oils*
   — Buchu
   — Oil of Cubel
   — Sandalwood oil
10. *Aldehyde group*
    — Hexamine

11. *Heavy metals*
    — Mercurochrome
    — Silver nitrate

3. Anti-diuretics

These are the drugs which diminish formation of urine either at glomerular or at tubular level

Classification

1. ***Drugs increasing renal tubular reabsorption***

    A. Drugs acting directly
    — Posterior pituitary extract
    — Vasopressin – 0.5 ml/alternate day to 1.0 ml t.d.s. (for Diabetes insipidus)

    B. Drugs acting indirectly by releasing ADH from posterior pituitary
    — Morphine
    — Apomorphine
    — Dimercaprol
    — Barbiturates

2. *Drugs decreasing glomerular filtration*
   A. Hypotensives
      — Hexamethonium
      — Mecamylamine
      — Pempidine
   B. Renal vasoconstriction
      — Adrenaline
      — Digitoxin in toxic doses
      — Morphine
   C. Purgatives (Act by producing dehydration)
      — Magnesium sulfate
      — Rhubarb
      — Jalap.

CHAPTER VII
ANTI-HISTAMINICS

1. *Ethylene diamines*
   — Mepyramine – 50-200 mg
   — Halopyramine (Synopen)
   — Tripelennamine (Pyribenzamine) – 25-50 mg b.d.
   — Meclizine – 25-50 mg
   — Chlorothen – 25 mg b.d.
   — Thonzylamine – 25-100 mg b.d.
2. *Monoamines (X—C)*
   — Pheniramine (Avil) – 25-50 mg b.d.
   — Chlorpheniramine – 8-12 mg b.d.
   — Brompheniramine – 4 mg t.d.s.
3. *Ethanolamines (X= O)*
   — Diphenhydramine (Benadryl) – 25-50 mg b.d. orally
   — Bromdiphenhydramine (Ambodryl) 25 mg b.d. orally

4. *Cyclizine derivatives*
   — Antazoline (Antistine) – Nasal sol. 5 mg/ml
   — Phenindamine – 10-25 mg t.d.s.
   — Cyclizine – 50 mg t.d.s.
   — Chlorcyclizine – 25-50 mg t.d.s.
5. *Miscellaneous*
   — Cyproheptadine (Periactin) – 4-20 mg/day
   — Mebhydrolin (Mebryl).

CHAPTER VIII
DRUGS ACTING ON UTERUS

1. *Oxytoxic drugs:* They increase the myometrial contraction
   — Oxytocin – 3-10 units I/M (0.3-1.0 ml)
   — Syntocinon
   — Ergometrine – 0.2 mg I/M or 0.5 mg orally
   — Methyl ergometrine – 0.2 mg I/M or I/V
   — Spartine sulfate – One ml I/M (150 mg)
   — Prostaglandins
   — Quinine ⎤ Not used clinically
   — Drastic purgatives ⎦
2. *Uterine relaxants*
   (a) Acting directly
   — Progesterone
   — Nitrites
   — Papaverine

(b) Adrenergic drugs
- Adrenaline
- Ephedrine
- Isoxuprine

(c) Cholinergic blocking drugs
- Atropine – 0.6 mg
- C.N.S. depressants
- Morphine – 15 mg I/M or I/V
- Pethidine – 100 mg I/M

(d) Non-steroidal ovarian hormones
- Luturin
- Releasin.

CHAPTER IX
DRUGS ACTING ON EYE

A. *Mydriatics :* These drugs dilate the pupil. They are classified as per their mode of action.
1. *Parasympatholytic drugs*
   — Atropine
   — Hyoscine
   — Homatropine
   — Cyclopentolate
2. *Sympathomimetic drugs*
   — Ephedrine – 0.5-3.0%
   — Amphetamine
   — Phenylephrine – 1-2%
3. *General anaesthetics*

B. *Myotics:* These are the drugs which constrict the pupil.
1. *Parasympathomimetic drugs*
   — Pilocarpine

- Physostigmine
- Methacholine
- Neostigmine
- Carbachol
2. *Sympatholytic drugs*
   - Dibenamine
3. *Other drugs*
   - Opium
- General anaesthetics (2nd and 4th stage)

C. *Drugs affecting accommodation*
   1. *Cycloplegics or drugs which paralyse accommodation*
      - Atropine – 0.5 – 1.0%
      - Hyoscine
      - Homatropine – 2%
   2. *Drugs which produce spasm of accommodation*
      - Pilocarpine

— Eserine
D. Drugs affecting intraocular tension
 1. *Drugs decreasing I/O tension*
    — Pilocarpine – 2% sol
    — Carbachol – 1.5% sol
    — Physostigmine – 0.5% sol
    — Acetazolamide (Diamox) – 250 mg tab. once daily
 2. *Drugs increasing I/O tension*
    — Atropine – 0.5-1% sol
    — Hyoscyamine
    — Hyoscine
    — Nitrites.

CHAPTER X
HAEMOPOIETIC SYSTEM

Classification of Drugs used in Anaemias

I. *Haematinics*
   — Iron and its salts
   (*a*) *Oral preparations*
   — Ferrous sulphate – 200-600 mg/day
   — Ferrous gluconate – 300 mg – 1.2 gm/daily
   — Ferrous lactate
   — Reduced iron
   (*b*) *Parenteral preparations*
   (*i*) *I/M*
   — Iron Dextran injection – 50-100 mg I/M daily
   — Iron Sorbitex injection (Jectofer) – 100 mg I/M daily
   — Green ferric amm. citrate

- Ferrous gluconate
- Iron adenylate
- Iron polyisomattose

(ii) I/V
- Iron Dextran injection
- Copper
- Cobalt
- Pyridoxine
- Riboflavin
- Protein

II. *Maturation factors*
- Vit B_{12} (Cyanocobalamine) – 500-1000 µg/day
- Vit B_{12} with intrinsic factor concentrate
- Liver injection one U.S.P. unit daily
- Folic acid
  - Tab. 5-20 mg/day
  - Inj.
- Folinic acid (Citrovorum factor)

Classification of Anticoagulants

I. *Heparin – Heparin sodium injection*
— 100-150 mg I/V six hourly (100 mg = 10,000 units)

II. *Oral anti-coagulants*

(a) *Coumarin derivatives*
— Dicumaral – 600 mg/day, maintenance dose 50-100 mg/day
— Liquamar – Loading dose 30 mg, maintenance dose 4 mg daily
— Acchocoumaral (Syntron) Loading dose 16-28 mg, maintenance dose 6 mg
— Warfarin sodium – 25-50 mg orally twice a week

(b) *Indendione derivatives*
— Phenindione (Danilene) – Initial dosage 200-300 mg/day, maintenance dosage 50-100 mg/day
— Diphenadione (Dipaxin) – Initial dose 30 mg, 2nd day 10-15 mg, maintenance dose 2.5-5 mg/day

— Anisinidione (Miradon) — 1st day – 300 mg
2nd day – 200 mg
3rd day – 100 mg
Maintenance dose – 75-100 mg/day

Drugs affecting platelet junction

Drugs inhibiting platelet aggression

— Aspirin
— Sulfinpyrazone
— Dipyridamole
— Dextran 40

COAGULANTS

A. Local Haemostatics

I. Physical agents

— Application of pressure or cold heat
— Oxidized cellulose
— Absorbable gelatin sponges
— Fibrin foam

II. *Astringents*
- Alum
- Ferrir chloride
- Tannic acid

III. *Drugs promoting the natural process of coagulation*
- Snake venoms
- Trypsin
- Staphylocoagulase
- Thrombin solution
- Fibrin

B. Systemic Haemostatics
- Vitamin K
- Anti-haemophilic globulin
- Fresh whole blood transfusion
- Calcium gluconate
- Adrenochrome monosemicarbazone
- Vitamin C
- Congo Red
- E-aminocaproic acid.

CHAPTER XI
DRUGS USED IN GOUT

I. *Drugs used in Acute Gout*

— Colchicine 4-8 mg [Start 1 mg orally and increase by 0.5-1 mg two hourly till relief is obtained]

— Demecolcine
— Phenylbutazone – 600-800 mg/day orally
— Cortisone
— Corticotrophin
— Indomethacin (Indocid) – 50-100 mg/day orally

II. *Drugs used in Chronic Gout (Uricosuric Agents)*

— Probenecid (Benemide) – 1-2 gm/day
— Salicylates
— Sulfinpyrazone (Anturan) – 100-400 mg/day orally
— Phenylbutazone (Butazolidin) 300-600 mg/day orally

- Cortisone
- Corticotrophin
- Cinchophen

III. *Inhibiting Uric Acid Synthesis*
- Allopurinol – 200-600 mg/day orally

DRUGS USED IN RHEUMATOID ARTHRITIS

I. *Anti-inflammatory*
- Salicylates, phenylbutazone: 100-300 mg/day orally
- Indomethacine – 25 mg t.d.s.
- Fenamate compounds: Ibuprofen (200-400 mg t.d.s.), Ketoprofen, Naproxen: 250 mg b.d.
- Anthranilates: Mefenamic acid
- Prednisone – 5-10 mg/day
- ACTH

II. *Gold salts:* Sodium aurothiomalate. Myochrysine 10 mg, 1st week, 25 mg, 2nd week later 50 mg weekly (I.M)

III. *Antimalarials:* Chloroquin, Hydrochloroquin 200 mg b.d.

IV. *d-penicillomine 250 mg b.d.*
V. *Immunosuppressive compounds: Alkylating agents.*

ANTISEPTICS AND DISINFECTANTS

1. *Acids:* Boric acid, Benzoic acid, Salicylic acid, Mandelic acid, Nalidixic acid
2. *Alkali:* Sodium hydroxide
3. *Alcohol:* Ethanol (70%)
4. *Aldehyde:* Formaldehyde, Methenamine
5. *Halogens:* Tr. Iodine, Iodoform, Bleaching powder, Chloramine
6. *Phenols:* Phenol, Cresol, Chlorcresol, Hexachlorophene
7. *Metals:* Silver nitrate, Silver chloride, Mercuric oxide, Mercurochrome, Mercuric chloride
8. *Dyes:* Crystal violet, Acriflavin, Pyridium
9. *Surfactants:*
    (a) *Anionic:* Soap, Sod. lauryl sulphate
    (b) *Catornic:* Cetyl pyridinum, Benzalkonium

10. *Miscellaneous:* Sulpher, Dequadin, Nitrofurans, Sandalwood oil, Clove oil
11. *Physical agents:* Ultraviolet rays, Autoclaving, Heating

VOLATILE OILS

I. *Those which act as counter-irritants:*
   1. Turpentine
   2. Camphor
   3. Menthol
   4. Mustard
   5. Oil of Eucalyptus
   6. Capsicum

II. *Those which act as carminatives:*
   1. Ajowan
   2. Oil of cassia
   3. Ginger
   4. Cardamom
   5. Nutmeg
   6. Oil of pudina
   7. Dill
   8. Pepermint oil

III. *Those which act as Anthelminthics:*
   1. Oil of chenopodium
   2. Turpentine
   3. Thymol

108 | *Classification of Drugs*

    IV. *Those which act as disinfectants:*
        1. Eucalyptus oil   2. Cinnamon
        3. Clove
    V. *Those which act as respiratory tract antiseptics*
        1. Creosote   2. Eucalyptus oil
    VI. *Those which act as urinary tract antiseptics*
        1. Sandal wood oil
        2. Cubeb
    VII. *Nauseants*
        1. Asafoetida
        2. Valerian

ANTI-PRURITICS

    I. *Anti-Histaminics*—orally
        1. Promethazine (Phenergan)
        2. Chlorpheniramine (Piriton) used orally
        3. Methdilazine (Dilosyn)
    II. *Local anaesthetics*
    III. *Calamine lotion*

IV. Camphor and menthol
V. Crotomiton oil
VI. Phenol (in lotion form)
VII. Alkaline bath (with sodium bicarbonate)
VIII. Evaporating lotions containing alcohol

SCLEROSING AGENTS

(Used in treatment of varicose veins)
1. Ethanolamine oleate
2. Sodium morrhuate
3. Injection of Quinine et urethane
4. Sodium linoleate
5. Oily phenol injection (5% soln). Used in treatment of haemorrhoids

KERATOLYTIC AGENTS

1. Salicylic acid
2. Dithranol
3. Lactic acid

EMOLLIENTS

1. Woolfat
2. Lanolin
3. Almond oil
4. Olive oil
5. Cotton seed oil
6. Liquid paraffin

BLOOD CHOLESTEROL REDUCING AGENTS

1. Clofibrate (Atromid S) – 1.5-2.5 gm/day orally
2. Nicotinamide – 3.6 gm/day orally
3. Dextro-thyroxine – 5-6 mg/day orally
4. Oestrogens
5. Triparanol – 250 mg/day orally
6. Unsaturated fats
7. Cholestyramine – 12 gm day orally

INSECTICIDES

1. *Natural substances*
   — Pyrethrum
   — Rotenone
2. *Chlorinated hydrocarbons*
   — Gamma benzene hexachloride
   — Endrin
3. *Organophosphorus compounds*
   — Malathion
   — Diazinon
   — Parathion
   — TEPP.

CHAPTER-XII
ENDOCRINOLOGY

Pituitary Hormone

(a) *Posterior pituitary*
   1. Oxytocin
   2. Vasopressin

(b) *Anterior pituitary (Important hormones are):*
   1. A.C.T.H.
   2. Growth hormone
   3. Folicular stimulating hormone (FSH)
   4. Luteinising hormone (LH)
   5. Thyroid stimulating hormone (TSH)
   6. Parathyroid stimulating hormone
   7. Prolactin

Thyroid Hormone Preparations

1. Thyroid extract – 60-180 mg/daily

2. Thyroglobulin
3. Sodium levothyroxine – 0.2-0.4 mg/day
4. Sodium liothyronine
5. Lyotrix

Anti-thyroid Drugs

I. Drugs interfering with trapping, i.e. blocking the iodide concentrating mechanism:
— Thiocyanate perchlorates

II. Drugs interfering with synthesis of hormone:

A.
— Thiourea
— Thiouracil
— Propyl thiouracil – 100-350 mg/day
— Methyl thiouracil – 50 mg. q.i.d.

B. *Imidazole derivatives*
— Methimazole
— Carbimazole

C. *Aniline derivatives*
   — Sulfonamides
   — Paraminobenzoic acid

D. *Polyhydric phenols*
   — Resorcinol

III. *Drugs which interfere with release of thyroid hormone*
   — Pot. iodide – 120-180 mg/day orally
   — Lugol's iodine – 1.5 ml/day orally

IV. *Drugs which destroy the thyroid gland:*
   — Radio active iodine
   I^{131}
   I^{130}
   I^{132}
   I^{128}
   I^{129}
   I^{125}

Classification of corticosteroids

I. *Glucocorticoids*

(a) *Natural*

— Hydrocortisone
- orally same as cortisone
- 0.5-2.5% oint locally
- 25 mg/ml for intra-articular use

— Cortisone– 25 mg q.i.d. for 4-5 days and then tapered gradually

(b) *Synthetic*

— Prednisolone
— Prednisone
  5 mg q.i.d. × 4-5 days and then tapered gradually

— Methyl prednisolone 16-20 mg daily
— Triamcinolone – 2-15 mg daily
— Paramethasone – 4-8 mg daily
— Dexamethasone – 1.5-3.0 mg daily 0.5-1% ophtha sol.
— Betamethasone – 1.2-3.6 mg/day. Maintenance dose – 0.6-3.0 mg daily

II. *Mineralocorticoids*
Natural – Aldosterone
Synthetic—
- Desoxy cortisone acetate – 1-3 mg/day
- Fludrocortisone – 0.1-0.3 mg/day
- Fluocortolone hexanoate

ANTI-DIABETIC AGENTS

I. *Insulin*
1. Soluble insulin (Short acting)
2. Protamine zinc insulin ⎤
3. Globin zinc insulin   ⎬ Retard insulins
4. Isophane insulin   ⎦
5. Insulin zinc suspensions (Lente insulins)
   - Insulin lente
   - Insulin semilente
   - Insulin ultralente
6. Actrapid ⎤ Purified insulins
7. Rapitard ⎦

II. *Oral Hypoglycaemic Drugs*
   (a) <u>Sulphonyl ureas:</u> (given orally)
      1. Tolbutamide (Rastinon) – 0.5-2 gm/day (in 1-4 doses)
      2. Chlorpropamide (Diabenese) – 100-500 mg in single dose
      3. Glibenclamide (Daonil) – 5-20 mg/day orally in 2-3 divided doses
      4. Acetohexamide – 0.5-1.5 gm/day
      5. Glymidine – 1-2 gm/day
   (b) *Biguanide derivatives :* (given in 2-4 doses orally)
      1. Phenformin (DBI) – 50-200 mg/day
      2. Metformin – 50-200 mg/day

CLASSIFICATION OF OESTROGENS

I. *Natural*
 — Estradiol – 1-5 mg I/M
 — Estrone – 1-10 mg orally or 0.1-1.0 mg I/M
 — Estriol

II. *Semisynthetic*
 — Ethinyl estradiol – Maintenance dose 0.02-0.05 mg daily
 — Mestranol
 — Guinestrol

III. *Esters of Estradiol*
 — Estradiol benzoate
 — Estradiol dipropionate

- Estradiol cypionate

Conjugated steroids
- Estrine sulphate

Polymeric steroids
- Polyestradiol phosphate

IV. *Synthetic non-steroidal estrogens*
- Diethyl stilbesterol
- Dienestrol – 0.1-3.5 mg daily
- Benzestrol – 2.5-5.0 mg I/M or S/C once or twice a week
- Hexestrol – 2-3 mg orally daily. 0.2-1.0 mg as maintenance dose
- Promethestrol – 1 mg t.d.s. orally, 1 mg daily maintenance dose
- Chlorotrianisene – 12-24 mg daily orally
- Methallenestril – 6 mg daily x 3 weeks and 3 mg daily subsequently

Classification of Progesterones

I. Progesterone and derivatives
- Progesterone – 5 mg oily solution I/M, 5-10 mg oral tab
- Dydrogesterone – 5-10 mg daily from 5th to 25th day of menstrual cycle
- Hydroxy progesterone coproate
- Medroxy progesterone acetate – 10-30 mg/day orally or 100 mg I/M fortnightly
- Chlormadinone acetate
- Magestrol acetate

II. 17-ethinyl testosterone derivatives
- Dimethisterone

III. 19-Nortestosterone derivatives
- Norethynodrel – 2.5-10 mg/day orally
- Norethindrone
- Norethindrone acetate
- Ethyl diacetate
- Di-norgestrol

Classification of Androgens

I. *Natural*
   — Testosterone

II. *Esters of testosterone*
   — Testosterone propionate – 25 mg I/M
   — Testosterone cypionate – 50-100 mg/ml oily sol.
   — Testosterone enunthate – 20 mg I/M every fortnightly or 3rd weekly

III. *Methylated testosterones*
   — Methyl testosterone – ointment 2-4 mg/gm 50-75 mg orally
   — Fluoxymesterone – 1.5 mg/day
   — Mesterolone

Anabolic steroids

I. *Orally available*
   — Ethyl estrenol (Maxibolin)
   — Methandrol (Stenediol)

- Methandrostenolone (Dianabol)
- Norethandrolone (Nilevar)
- Oxandrolone (Anavar)
- Oxymetholone (Adroyd Anadrol)
- Stanatine (Anabolax, Aondrolines Neodrol)
- Sianazolol (Winstrol)
- Testolactone (Teslac)

II. *Parenteral preparations (I/M)*
- Dromostanolone propionate (Drolban)
- Nandrolone decanoate (Decadurabolin)
- Nandrolone phenpropionate (Durabolin).

CHAPTER XIII
CHEMOTHERAPY

Drugs used in Bacterial Infection
1. Sulfonamides
2. Antibiotics
3. Anti-tubercular drugs
4. Anti-leprosy drugs

1. Sulfonamides
(i) Short acting sulfonamides
- Sulfadiazine – 2 gm stat then 1 gm 4-6 hourly
- Sulfamethizol – 1 gm 6 hourly
- Sulfamerazine – 2 gm stat then 1 gm 4-6 hourly
- Sulfamethazine
- Sulfadimidine 2 gm stat then 1 gm 4-6 hourly
- Sulfasomidine – 1 gm 6 hourly

(ii) *Locally acting sulfonamides (Absorbed very less)*
  — Sulfaguanidine
  — Pthalyl sulfathiazole – 1 gm six hourly
  — Pthalyl sulfacetamide
  — Succinyl sulfathiazol 2-3 gm 4 hourly

(iii). *Long acting sulfonamides*
  — Sulfaphenazole (orisul) – 2 gm stat then 1 gm 12 hourly
  — Sulfadimethoxine (Madribon) – 1 gm stat then 0.5 gm/day
  — Sulfamethoxypyridazine (Lederkyn) – 1 gm stat then 0.5 gm/day

2. Antibiotics
  — Classification of antibiotics

(i) Antibacterial antibiotics

1. Penicillins
   A. *Parenterally used Penicillins*
   - *(i) Short acting*
     - Sodium Penicillin G
     - Potassium Penicillin G
     - Oxacillin sodium
   - *(ii) Long acting*
     - Procaine Penicillin G – 400,000 I.U. I/M daily
     - PAM (Penicillin with Aluminium monosterate)
     - Benzathine Penicillin 1.2 mega unit I/M fortnightly

   B. *Orally used Penicillins*
   - Phenoxymethyl Penicillin 250-500 mg 6 hourly
   - Cloxacillin – 250-500 mg 6 hourly
   - Oxacillin – 500 mg orally 6 hourly
   - Nafcillin 500 mg I/M 6 hourly, 250-500 mg orally 6 hourly

C. *Penicillinase resistant Penicillins*
- Methicillin – 1 gm I/M 4-6 hourly
- Cloxacillin
- Oxacillin – 500 mg 6 hourly orally
- Nafcillin – 250-500 mg orally 6 hourly
- Ampicillin – 250-500 mg 6 hourly

D. *Broad spectrum Penicillins*
- Ampicillin 250-500 mg I/M or orally 6 hourly
- Hetacillin
- Carbenicillin

E. *Acid resistant Penicillins*
- Phenoxymethyl Penicillin V – 125-250 mg orally
- Phenoxyethyl Penicillin
- Phenoxypropyl Penicillin
- Phenoxybenzyl Penicillin

2. **Cephalosporines**
   - Cephadrine
   - Cephalthin
3. **Erythromycin group**
   - Erythromycin estolate
   - Erythromycin stearate
4. **Tetracycline group**
   - Tetracyclines
   - Demeclocycline
   - Methacycline
   - Doxycycline
5. **Chloramphenicol**
6. **Aminoglycosides**
   - Streptomycin
   - Neomycin
   - Kanamycin

7. **Polymyxin**
   — Polymyxin B Sulphate
   — Colistin

Penicillins

   (ii) *Anti-viral and anti-rickettsial antibiotics*
   — Tetracyclines
   — Chloramphenicol

   (iii) *Anti-fungal antibiotics*
   — Griseofulvin – 500 mg daily in divided doses
   — Amphotericin B – 50 mg daily in I/V transfusion
   — Nystatin – 500,000 units t.d.s. orally

   (iv) *Anti-amoebic antibiotics*
   — Tetracycline
   — Paromomycin

- Fumagillin – 30-60 mg daily in divided doses
  - (v) *Anti-neoplastic antibiotics*
    - Chromomycin
    - Actinomycin D – 0.2-0.5 mg I/V
    - Mitomycin
    - Azaserine – 2.5 mg/kg orally daily
    - Adriamycin

3. **Antitubercular Drugs**
   1. ***Drugs used as first line of treatment***
      - (i) *Antibiotics*
        - Streptomycin – 1 gm I/M daily
        - Rifampicin – 450-600 mg/day orally
      - (ii) *Other chemotherapeutic agents*
        - PAS (Paraminosalicylic acid) – 12-15 gm daily
        - Sodium aminosalicylic acid

- Calcium aminosalicylic acid
- Isoniazide 300 mg daily
- Ethambutol – 25 mg/kg body wt/day

2. *Drugs used as second line of treatment*
   (a) *Antibiotics*
      - Viomycin – 2 gm I/M twice a day
      - Kanamycin – 1 gm I/M daily
      - Cycloserine – 0.5-1.0 gm/day
      - Rifamycin
   (b) *Other chemotherapeutic agents*
      - Thiosemicarbazone
      - Ethionamide 500-1000 mg/day orally
      - Pyrazinamide 40 mg/kg/day orally

4. Anti-leprosy Drugs

1. *Naturally occurring products*
   - Oil of chaul moorga
   - Oil of hydnocarpus

2. *Sulfones*
   — Dapsone – 10-50 mg biweekly gradually in increasing doses upto 100-200 mg biweekly.
   — Sulfetrone (Solapsone) – 1.5 gm/day × 7 days then increase by 1-2 gm/week, maximum upto 6-10 gm/day
   — Sulfoxone
   — Glucosulfone

3. *Antibiotics*
   — Streptomycin
   — Paromomycin
   — Erythromycin
   — Fumagillin

4. *Thiourea compounds*
   — Thiambutosin – 1-3 gm/day, increase gradually by 500 mg/day

5. *Miscellaneous*
   — INH
   — Thiacetazone – 50 mg/day increase gradually upto 200 mg/day orally
   — Blofazimine

5 Drugs used for Syphilis

(i) *Antibiotics*
   — Penicillin – 600 mg I/M daily × 10 days
   — Benzathine penicillin – 1.2 million units I/M fortnightly
   Other antibiotics viz
   — Erythrocin ⎤
   — Tetracycline ⎥ 500 mg 6 hourly × 3 weeks used only if patient is sensitive to Penicillin
   — Chloramphenicol ⎦

(ii) *Arsenic compounds*
   — Arsphenamine
   — Oxophenarsine
   — Tryparsamide

(*iii*) *Iodides* – Potassium iodide

(*iv*) *Mercurials*
- Liq. hydrag perchlor
- Mercurous and mercuric oxide lotion used locally

(v) *Bismuth salts*
- Bismuth oxychloride
- Bismuth salicylase

6. **Anti-viral Drugs**
   - Idoxyuridine
   - Adamantanamine
   - Interferon
   - Methisazone
   - Chloramphenicol
   - Tetracyclines
   - Sulfonamides

7. **Anti-neoplastic Drugs**
   (a) *Drugs used in Lymphoblastic Leukaemias*
      (i) *Acute*
         — 6 mercaptopurines – 2.5 mg/kg/day orally
         — Vincristine
         — Methotrexate – 2.5-10 mg/day orally
         — Asparaginase
         — Anti-lymphocytic serum
         — Corticosteroids
      (ii) *Chronic*
         — Chlorambucil (Leukeran) – 0.1-0.2 mg/kg/day orally
         — Cyclophosphamide (Endoxon) 2-8 mg/kg/day orally or I/V
   (b) *Drugs used in Myeloid Leukaemias*
      (i) *Acute*
         — Daunorubicin

- 6 Mercaptopurine
- Asparaginase
- Cytosine arabinoside

(ii) *Chronic*
- Busulfan (Myleran) – 4-6 mg/day orally
- Hydroxy urea

(c) **Drugs used in Hodgkin's Disease**
- Procarbazine
- Mustine hydrochloride
- Cyclophosphamide – 2-8 mg/kg/day orally or I/V
- Vinblastine

(d) **Drugs used in Chorio Carcinoma**
- Methotrexate – 2.5-10 mg/day orally
- Vinblastine
- Actinomycin D

8. Chemotherapy of Helminthic Infections

Anti-helminthic drugs are those which are used to remove or kill the worms infesting the body.

(i) *Drugs used against hookworm*
- Bephenium hydroxynaphthoate (Alcopar) – single 5 gm dose
- Tetrachlorethylene – 3-4 ml
- Carbon tetrachloride – 1.5-3.0 ml
- Hexyl resorcinol
- Oil of Chenopodium – 1.5-3.0 ml
- Thiabendazole (Mintezol) – 25 mg/kg/orally/day
- Mebendazone – 100 mg b.d. × 3 days
- Tetramizole (Decaris) – 150 mg orally (single dose at bed time)

(ii) *Drugs used against roundworm*
- Piperazine citrate – 50 mg/kg body wt average 3.5 gm single dose × 2 days
- Mebendazole – 100 mg b.d. × 3 days
- Diethylcarbamazine

- Hexyl resorcinol
- Santonin – 50-200 mg orally
- Oil of chenopodium – 1.5-3.0 ml

(iii) *Drugs used against threadworm (Entrobiasis)*
- Piperazine citrate – 2 gm daily × 3 weeks
- Hexyiresorcinol
- Promethazine
- Pyrvinium (Vanquin) – 5 mg/kg body wt
- Mebendazole – 100 mg single dose
- Gention and crystal violet
- Garlic
- Oxytetracyclin

(iv) *Drugs used against whipworm (Trichuriasis)*
- Hexylresorcinol
- Tetrachlorethylene
- Oil of chenopodium
- Cyanine dye

- Thiabendazole (Mintezol) – 50 mg/kg/day
- Mebendazole – 100 mg b.d × 3 days

(v) *Drugs used against tapeworm*
- Mepacrine – 800 mg total dose orally
- Chloroquine
- Filix mass – 1-5 gm
- Tin compounds
- Yomesan (Niclosamide) – 1-2 gm orally

(vi) *Drugs used for Amoebiasis*

(a) Ipecacuanha drugs
- Emetine hydrochloride – 30-60 mg/day I/M × 10 days
- Dehydroemetine hydrochloride – 1 mg/kg × 10 days I/M

(b) 8 Amino-quinoline derivatives
- Di-iodohydroxy quinoline – 1-2 mg/day × 3 weeks

— Iodochlorhydroxyquinoline – 500 mg – 1 gm/day × 2 weeks

(c) Aminoquinoline derivatives

— Chloroquin – 600 mg/day × 2 days (Loading dose), 300 mg/day × 3 weeks

(d) Arsenic compounds

— Acetarsol – 500 mg/day × 10 days

— Carbarson – 0.5 gm/day × 10 days

(e) Nitro-imidazole derivatives

— Metronidazole – 2 tab thrice daily × 10 days (600-2400 mg/day)

(f) Miscellaneous

— Phanquone (Entobex) – 300 mg/day orally

— Furamide – 1.5 gm/day × 10 days

— Tetracycline

— Paromomycin – 25 mg/kg/day orally

(vii) *Drugs used against giardiasis*
- Metronidazole
- Chloroquine
- Mepacrine
- Acetarsol
- Furazolidine (Furoxone)
- Phanquone (Entobex)

(viii) *Drugs used against Trichomoniasis*

1. *Drugs used locally*
   - Acetarsol
   - Carbarsol
   - Silver salts
   - Boric acid

2. *Drugs used systemically*
   - Metronidazole – 2 tablets thrice daily × 7 days

(ix) *Anti-malarial drugs*
   1. *Cinchona alkaloids*
      — Quinine 300-600 mg/day
      — Quinidine
      — Cinchonine
   2. *4-amino quinolines*
      — Chloroquin – 4 tab stat (150 mg base) after 6 hours 1 b.d. × 3 days
      — Amodiaquin (Camoquin) 600 mg as single dose
   3. *8-amino quinolines*
      — Pamaquin – 10-20 mg/day
      — Pentaquin – 30 mg/day
      — Primaquin – 10-15 mg/day
   4. *Biguanide derivatives*
      — Paludrin
   5. *Acridine derivatives*
      — Mepacrine – 200-500 mg/day.